THIS BOOK BELONGS TO

www.ingramcontent.com/pod-product-compliance
Lightning Source LLC
Chambersburg PA
CBRC091537260326
41914CB00022B/1648

9781953987143